HEALING BEYOND *THE* HUSTLE

How Work Tried to Break Me – and Failed

LATOYA·MONROE-LOVE

Table of Contents

Acknowledgments

First and foremost, I give honor and glory to God, who is the head of my life and the guiding hand behind every word written in this book. Without His grace, I would not have the strength to share my story or the courage to walk in my purpose.

To my husband, thank you for standing beside me through every high and low. Your unwavering support, patience, and love gave me the courage to keep moving forward when I felt like giving up. You are my safe place, and you are my reminder that I am never alone in this journey.

To my children, you are my heart. Watching you grow gives me purpose beyond measure. You are my daily reminder of why I choose healing over pain and peace over chaos. I pray this book becomes part of the legacy I leave for you.

To my church family at The Dwelling Place, thank you for being my spiritual anchor. Your prayers, encouragement, and covering carried me through some of my darkest seasons and reminded me that God's light always shines brighter than any storm.

To every survivor, advocate, and soul who has been silenced by toxic workplaces or broken systems, I wrote this for you. May you find healing, validation, and the power to rise again. Your pain is not the end of your story.

To those who poured into me with love, truth, and correction, you helped shape the woman behind these pages. Thank you for speaking life into me, reminding me of my strength, and holding me accountable to the vision God placed in my heart.

To my best friends, thank you for seeing me, encouraging me, and reminding me of my voice when I was close to giving up. Your love and support inspired this book and gave me the push to turn my pain into purpose.

Finally, to every reader who holds this book in your hands, thank you. By choosing to spend time with my story, you've become part of my healing journey. I pray these words meet you where you are and encourage you to believe that healing beyond purpose is not only possible, but it is also waiting for you too.

Dedication

This book is dedicated to my husband and children whose love carried me through seasons of brokenness and whose lives were impacted by the battles I faced in toxic workplaces. You endured the weight of my pain and stood with me in the storm. It is also dedicated to every survivor whose family, spirit, and future were shaken by unjust systems. May these words remind you that healing is not just for you. It is for those who love you and for the generations that follow.

INTRODUCTION

Why This Book Exists

I didn't set out to write a book about workplace trauma. In fact, for a long time, I didn't even have the words for what I was experiencing. I just knew I was tired—not the kind of tired a weekend off could fix but the bone-deep exhaustion that seeps into your spirit and makes you question everything.

I thought that was just "the grind." I thought everyone was supposed to feel like that if they wanted to succeed. I told myself to push through. Smile more. Work harder. I am grateful I even had a job.

However, the truth is that no amount of hustle can heal an environment that is harming you, and no paycheck is worth your peace, your health, or your soul.

I wrote this book because too many of us have been told to just "be resilient" instead of being asked why we have to be resilient in the first place. We've been conditioned to normalize stress, hide our pain, and measure our worth in productivity.

This is my story, but it's also a mirror.

You'll see yourself in these pages if you've ever stayed in a job that drained you because you felt trapped, silenced your voice to keep the peace, or doubted your worth because of how you were treated at work.

In these chapters, I'll share:

- What workplace trauma really looks like (and why it's more common than we think).
- How to recognize the signs before you reach your breaking point.
- The tools I used to reclaim my stability, protect my boundaries, and rebuild my life.
- Why leadership has the power to either harm or heal and what must change at the top.

This isn't just a survival guide. It's an invitation:

- To choose yourself.
- To leave behind the belief that suffering is part of the job description.
- To see your value beyond what you produce.
- To step into life beyond the hustle.

You don't need permission to heal.

You just need the courage to start, but the truth is that workplace trauma doesn't end when you clock out. It follows you home. It seeps into family dinners, quiet nights, and even the way you parent. My exhaustion wasn't just mine. My family carried it too. They saw the pieces of me that work had broken. They felt the heaviness in the air, and sometimes, they absorbed my silence or my pain.

This book is not just about what happened to me inside the workplace, but it is also about how the ripple effects touched my home, my marriage, and my children because when a system harms one person, it rarely harms them alone.

CHAPTER 1

Before the Healing Began

Before the healing began, life had already taught me about survival. I grew up in an environment where stability was rare, and loss was familiar. The sound of gunshots, the sight of drug activity, and the quiet moments of fear all became the backdrop of my childhood. I remember the sudden panic when drug dealers ran into our home, hiding from the police. Their presence turned my safe space into a place of chaos. I remember the grief and shock I felt when my uncle was murdered by his own family. Death was so close that it felt like it could touch anyone at any moment. Most of the time, all I knew was fear and worry. Those early years shaped me to be strong, resourceful, and independent, but they also taught me to carry far more than any child should—the unspoken responsibility to manage emotions that weren't mine and protect others while quietly shielding myself.

When I became a mother, my sense of responsibility doubled. Suddenly, I was not only accountable for my own survival, but I was also responsible for nurturing tiny humans who relied on me to feel safe in a world that often felt unsafe. I fought to create a different life for my children—a life with safety, love, and opportunities I had to imagine for myself. This meant working long hours, advocating tirelessly, and showing up, even when exhaustion made my bones ache. It meant putting their needs first, and often, I had to put mine last.

For years, I lived in a rhythm of overwork and underrest. I balanced school assignments, multiple jobs, and motherhood while carrying anxiety, depression, and guilt like hidden baggage I couldn't set down. Every day was a marathon of "get it done" and "keep going," with no pause to ponder, *How am I really doing?*

What I didn't know then was that the workplace—the place I thought would give me purpose, stability, and respect—could also become a source of harm. The emotional exhaustion I felt wasn't just from my personal life; it was compounded by environments that demanded more than they gave and applauded resilience but never questioned why I had to be so resilient in the first place. Small slights, microaggressions, and the constant tension of having to perform perfectly became normalized. I started to think that being constantly on edge, always anxious, was simply part of being a "good worker" and a "good mother."

Back then, I didn't have the language for workplace trauma. I didn't recognize the subtle ways my environment chipped away at my confidence, energy, and peace of mind. I thought it was just hard work, just ambition, and just life. I didn't realize that dread in the pit of my stomach before going to work, the sleepless nights worrying about making mistakes, and the quiet voice inside me begging for rest were all warning signs.

Looking back, I see now that my healing didn't begin when I left a toxic job or when I finally spoke up. It began the moment I started to recognize my worth—outside of my work, outside of my roles, and outside of what anyone else expected of me.

This chapter is about that time before the healing began—the time when I was surviving, not yet free, and carrying burdens silently while believing I was alone in them. It's about acknowledging that struggle because before we heal, we must first remember what it felt like to be unhealed.

Reflection for the Reader:

Think about your own "before." What patterns, pressures, or pain did you accept as normal? What voices inside or outside told you to keep going, even when your body and mind were exhausted? Awareness is the first crack in the wall that keeps you trapped. Naming what was unhealthy and what was overwhelming is the first step toward reclaiming your freedom.

CHAPTER 2

The Breaking Point

There comes a moment when the body and mind refuse to keep carrying what the spirit can no longer bear. For me, that moment came quietly, not in an explosion, but in a slow, suffocating realization—*I can't keep doing this.*

I had been working in human services for years, pouring myself into helping others. On paper, it looked noble. It was draining me. The work was relentless—long hours, short staffing, constant crises. I was often placed in environments that were physically unsafe and emotionally volatile. I remember walking into my office some mornings feeling like I was stepping into a battlefield, but I had no armor on. My chest was tight, and my stomach was in knots.

I started waking up with headaches. My heart was racing before I even got out of bed. My patience was gone. My smile felt heavy. Small interactions, like clients lashing out or attacking me or my colleagues, left me drained. Sometimes, I had to restrain a client for minutes at a time, stopping briefly to stay in compliance. Restraints couldn't last more than fourteen and a half minutes—only to step right back in for another forty-five minutes. The management didn't support us the way we needed, and when staff called out from exhaustion, some were suspended without pay. I felt exhausted, and I was constantly on edge, like my body was running a marathon I couldn't finish.

Worse than the exhaustion was the isolation. When I spoke up about the pressure, the response was often, "That's just the job," as if my burnout was proof I wasn't tough enough rather than a signal that the system itself was broken. I began to feel invisible. I felt that my efforts went unnoticed, and my voice felt unheard. The weight of it slowly crushed me from the inside out.

That's when I began to understand the difference among stress, burnout, and work trauma:

- Stress is the body's natural response to challenges; it comes and goes.
- Burnout is when prolonged stress leaves you physically, mentally, and emotionally depleted.
- Work trauma is deeper. It's when the workplace itself becomes a source of harm, triggering feelings of fear, helplessness, or betrayal.

I wasn't just stressed. I wasn't even "just" burned out. I was experiencing trauma from the very place I had committed myself to serve.

The signs were there:

- Trouble sleeping—I felt this even when I was exhausted. I would lie awake at night, replaying every interaction, every missed deadline, and every moment I felt unseen.

- Emotional numbness—I felt like I was watching my life instead of living it. I laughed, and I smiled, but inside, I was empty.

- Dreading work—I felt this, not because it was hard, but because it felt unsafe—emotionally and sometimes physically.

I wasn't alone either. I later learned that workplace trauma impacts people across industries—healthcare workers, educators, retail employees, corporate professionals. Trauma doesn't care about your title; it cares about your environment.

The breaking point wasn't a single event. It was the accumulation of being undervalued, unheard, and overworked until the only option left was to choose myself. That choice felt terrifying, but it was the first step toward reclaiming my life. I remember sitting in my car one morning before heading into work, feeling like my chest would collapse. I realized I couldn't keep sacrificing my health, my spirit, or my peace. Saying "enough" wasn't easy, but it was necessary.

Reflection for the Reader:

Think about your own breaking point. Was it a single moment, or was it a slow build up over time? What signals did your body, mind, or spirit give you that you couldn't ignore? Recognizing these signs is not weakness; it's awareness. It is the first step toward setting boundaries and reclaiming your well-being.

CHAPTER 3

Know Your Rights, Your Voice: Empowering the Overwhelmed Worker

When you're caught in a toxic workplace, it's easy to believe you have no options. The environment convinces you that speaking up will cost you your job, your peace, or your reputation. I know that feeling well—the fear of rocking the boat, even when you're drowning.

Here's the truth; silence protects the system, not you.

For years, I didn't fully understand my workplace rights. I thought loyalty meant endurance, showing up no matter how harmful the conditions became. I didn't realize that my silence was costing me more than my comfort; it was costing me my health, my safety, and my sense of worth.

I used to often feel like my rights were being violated, so I spent a lot of time researching what was happening, making sure my rights as an employee weren't being ignored. They would ask for personal information that didn't seem necessary, and I felt they were doing whatever they wanted simply because they could. Most of the staff were too afraid of losing their jobs to question anything, signing everything without hesitation, but not me. Standing my ground was crucial, especially with all I was going through personally.

Knowing your rights changes everything. It gives you the language to name what's happening, the power to set boundaries, and the confidence to demand fair treatment. It also protects you from internalizing harm as "just part of the job."

Your Universal Rights as a Worker

No matter what the industry, you have rights that are protected under law, and these rights exist to safeguard your well-being:

- The right to work in a safe and healthy environment
- The right to be free from harassment and discrimination
- The right to fair wages and pay transparency
- The right to reasonable accommodations for disabilities or health conditions
- The right to speak up about unsafe conditions without retaliation

Why This Knowledge Matters

When you don't know your rights, you're more vulnerable to exploitation. Toxic workplaces thrive on confusion; they benefit when employees feel replaceable and powerless.

Knowing your rights doesn't mean every battle will be easy, but it means you're no longer fighting blind. You can pause, take a breath, and respond from a place of clarity instead of fear. Knowing your rights is also how you take care of yourself—your energy, your health, and your peace of mind. Most people are scared to fight for their rights, but learning them is the first step toward empowerment.

Practical First Steps When You Feel Overwhelmed

1. **Pause Before Reacting** – When emotions are high, give yourself space to think before responding.

2. **Document Everything** – Keep detailed records of incidents, conversations, and dates.

3. **Review Your Employee Handbook** – This is your roadmap for company policies, procedures, and protections.

4. **Ask Questions** – If something doesn't feel right, clarify. You don't have to sign or agree blindly.

5. **Seek Outside Support** – Talk to HR, legal aid, or an employment rights advocate.

6. **Use Your Voice Strategically** – Decide when to speak up directly and when to escalate through proper channels.

7. **Protect Your Peace** – Not every fight is yours to fight. Choose the ones that matter most for your well-being.

Reflection for the Reader

- What rights do you need to learn more about in your current or past workplace?

- How could that knowledge have changed your choices?

- Are there moments when standing your ground could have protected your energy, health, or dignity?

Knowing your rights is more than a legal matter; it's a mental health matter. It's how you protect your energy, your dignity, and your ability to walk away when staying costs too much.

Resources for Knowing and Protecting Your Workplace Rights

Knowing your rights is one thing, but having access to resources that can guide and support you is just as important. Here are some trusted organizations and tools:

1. U.S. Department of Labor (DOL)

Website: www.dol.gov

- Provides information on workplace rights, including wages, safety, and working conditions.

- Offers guidance for filing complaints about labor law violations.

2. Equal Employment Opportunity Commission (EEOC)

Website: www.eeoc.gov

- Handles complaints about workplace discrimination based on race, color, religion, sex, national origin, age, disability, or genetic information.
- Offers tips for documenting incidents and filing claims.

3. National Employment Law Project (NELP)

Website: www.nelp.org

- Advocates for workers' rights and provides resources on wage theft, unemployment, and fair labor standards.

4. Legal Aid or Employment Rights Advocates

- Local legal aid organizations can help you understand your rights, review contracts, and even represent you if needed.
- Example: Search "[Your State] legal aid employment rights" to find resources nearby.

5. Your Employee Handbook and HR Department

- Always review your handbook for company policies and reporting procedures.
- HR is often the first internal resource for complaints or clarification.

6. Documenting Tools

- Keep a secure folder (digital or physical) with records of conversations, emails, and any incidents.
- Apps like Evernote, Google Drive, or even a dedicated journal can help organize evidence.

Tip: Even if you feel hesitant, **learning your rights and knowing where to turn** gives you power. You don't have to fight alone, and asking questions is a form of self-care.

CHAPTER 4

The Effects of Not Knowing Your Rights

Not knowing your workplace rights isn't just a gap in knowledge; it's a silent trap. It leaves you vulnerable, unsure, and more likely to accept treatment you don't deserve.

I've lived it. I've stayed in situations that chipped away at my self-worth because I didn't realize I had the authority to push back. Without that knowledge, you start to believe the problem is you.

The Emotional Toll

When you don't know your rights, the emotional weight grows heavy:

- You second-guess yourself constantly.
- You feel guilty for needing rest or asking for help.
- You normalize behavior that would shock you in any other context.

Shame creeps in, whispering that maybe you're just not strong enough. You start to shrink your voice to keep the peace, even as the cost to your mental health rises.

Action Tip: Take a moment to name your feelings. Ask yourself, *Is this guilt or is this a sign that my boundaries are being crossed?*

The Mental Fog

The stress of uncertainty creates a mental fog that clouds your judgment. You stop recognizing red flags because they've become part of the scenery. You tell yourself this is just how it is, even when your gut knows better.

This fog blurs the line between dedication and exploitation. It convinces you to push through exhaustion, accept unfair treatment, and overextend yourself for the sake of "being a team player."

Action Tip: Pause and record the patterns you notice. Writing them down can help separate your gut instinct from the pressure to conform.

The Career Consequences

Over time, the cost isn't just emotional; it's professional.

- You might stay in unsafe or unhealthy environments far longer than you should.
- You accept pay that doesn't match your skills or workload.

- You pass up promotions or opportunities because you don't believe you can negotiate for more.

Perhaps the most damaging effect is that you start to think that this is all you're worth.

The costs of silence ripple far beyond emotions, and they shape your career and self-perception.

Why Knowing Your Rights is a Form of Healing

When you understand your rights, you begin to rewrite the narrative. You stop blaming yourself for systems designed to protect employers more than employees. You see the bigger picture; your worth is not defined by how much you can endure.

This awareness doesn't just protect you in the workplace; it strengthens your sense of self in every area of life. Knowing your rights is not only legal protection, but it is also a form of self-care, boundary-setting, and reclaiming your voice.

Reflection for the Reader:

Think about a time when you didn't speak up because you didn't know you could. What would you do differently now with the knowledge you have? How can taking a stand for yourself—even in small ways—protect your peace and your future?

CHAPTER 5

The Trauma Bond

When you don't know your rights, you're left questioning yourself instead of questioning the system. That uncertainty doesn't just hold you back; it ties you down. Over time, it can create something even more dangerous than silence—a trauma bond.

For me, that bond seemed like convincing myself that the way I was working was okay because I needed to provide for my family. I told myself the long hours, the constant stress, and the lack of rest were just part of being responsible, but the truth was that it broke me.

Management reinforced that cycle by making me feel like taking time off was a weakness. If I even thought about rest, I worried I'd be written up or punished. I never once took a full week's vacation in over ten years of working at that company, not even to spend time with my children. What I thought was dedication was really burnout dressed up as loyalty.

Then came the breaking point. One of the most supportive and influential leaders in the company—someone almost everyone leaned on—was suddenly fired. Ninety percent of the staff was left in shock, and it shattered any illusion of stability I had left. That moment forced me to see how deep the trauma bond ran. It also became a turning point, one of the reasons I eventually stepped into becoming a behavioral specialist. I didn't want others to stay trapped in cycles that harmed them the way I once was harmed.

Trauma bonds don't look obvious from the outside. To others, it may seem like you're simply loyal, committed, or even thriving, but inside, you know the cost. You know the exhaustion of being torn between the hope that things will improve and the reality that they never do. That is the quiet prison of a trauma bond, and many of us, without realizing it, are living behind those invisible bars. Sometimes, the heaviest chains are invisible.

They don't rattle, and they don't clang, but they live inside of us, stitched into the way we hope, fear, and endure.

That's what a **trauma bond** is.

It's not love. It's not loyalty. It's survival. It's the tie that keeps you connected to the very place or person that is slowly draining you because leaving feels more dangerous than staying.

In a toxic workplace, a trauma bond can sound like this:

- "It's not that bad. I can handle it."
- "They've done worse, but they've also been kind."

- "If I leave, I might not find anything better."
- "I just need to push through."

I know those words. I've whispered them to myself.

I've stayed in jobs that hollowed me out because I thought loyalty meant sacrificing my peace. I confused endurance with strength. I convinced myself that pain was just the price of success.

What I didn't see at the time was how deeply the cycle had hooked me.

Why We Stay

Trauma bonds are powerful because they mix harm with hope. One day, your boss praises your hard work, and you feel seen. The next day, they belittle you, and you shrink. However, by then, you're already waiting for the next crumb of validation.

It's the push-and-pull that traps you. The unpredictability creates a false sense of "maybe tomorrow will be different." You hold on to the good days like lifelines, even as the bad days quietly erode your spirit.

This is how the cycle keeps spinning, not because you're weak but because you're human.

Breaking the Bond

Breaking free doesn't always look like slamming a door and never looking back. Sometimes, it starts with whispers of truth and small, steady steps.

Here's how that journey can look:

1. **Recognize the Pattern** – Say it out loud, "This is hurting me." Naming it is the first cut in the chain.

2. **Speak the Truth** – Tell your story to someone safe: a friend, a mentor, or even just yourself in a journal.

3. **Set Boundaries** – Decide what you will no longer accept and honor that decision.

4. **Build Support** – Surround yourself with people who remind you of your worth, especially when you forget.

5. **Plan Your Exit** – Whether you leave tomorrow or in a year, create a plan that protects your finances, your health, and your dignity.

Every small act of reclaiming yourself loosens the grip of the bond.

Why This Matters for Healing

When you break a trauma bond, you're not just leaving a toxic workplace; you're ending the cycle. You're refusing to carry those chains into the next job, the next relationship, or the next version of yourself.

Healing isn't about proving your endurance. It's about choosing your freedom.

Every time you choose yourself over fear, you reinforce this truth:

You are not replaceable. You are not disposable. You deserve better.

Reflection for the Reader:

Think about a time you stayed in a situation that was slowly breaking you. What kept you there? If you could go back, how would freedom have looked sooner?

Breaking the trauma bond was the first, most crucial step, but freedom isn't a single day or a single decision; it's a series of choices we make for ourselves. Sometimes, we make them quietly or boldly, and we make them every single day. Choosing yourself isn't about escaping harm; it's about building stability, reclaiming your identity, and learning what it truly means to thrive.

CHAPTER 6

How You Navigated Challenges and Found Stability

Choosing yourself is rarely a single decision; it's a series of small, steady choices that add up to freedom.

When I finally stepped away from a toxic work environment, it wasn't because I had everything figured out. It was because I knew staying there would cost me more than leaving. I was exhausted, mentally frayed, and physically worn down. My spirit had been sounding the alarm for months, and I could no longer ignore it.

The Role of Therapy and Self-Care

- Therapy became my lifeline. For the first time, I had a space where my feelings weren't minimized or dismissed. I learned how to name my emotions, set boundaries without guilt, and untangle my identity from my job title.

- Self-care shifted from being something I fit in if I had time to something I prioritized daily, even if I did it in small ways:
- Morning meditation instead of immediately checking my phone.
- Journaling to release thoughts instead of letting them spiral in my head.
- Taking walks without turning them into multitasking sessions.

Boundaries as a Form of Stability

One of the biggest lessons I learned was that stability isn't about keeping everything under control. It's about controlling what I allow into my space. Once I was able to see that, it helped me find balance.

That meant saying "no" more often, declining opportunities that would drain me, and choosing environments that valued me as a human being, not just a worker.

Practical Tips for Workplace Stability

If you're in the process of rebuilding, here are a few strategies that helped me:

1. **Time Management with Compassion** – Schedule your tasks but leave room for rest.

2. **Resilience through Reflection** – End your day by noting what went well, even if it's small.

3. **Peer Support** – Find coworkers or friends who understand your goals and will hold you accountable.

4. **Ongoing Learning** – Invest in professional development that aligns with your values.

5. **Clear Communication** – Speak your needs early instead of letting resentment build.

Why This Season Mattered

This period of my life taught me that healing isn't just about leaving something harmful; it's about building something healthy in its place. I began to see that personal healing could only go so far if workplaces remained toxic.

I realized I wasn't just interested in surviving my career; I wanted to change how workplaces functioned. That meant shifting the conversation from self-care to system care.

Family and Perspective

Once I left the job, I began seeing things differently. I noticed the path my children were going in, and I saw my husband going through the lack of love during the most needed time. My sons finally saw their mom at home, cooking dinner, spending time with them, and being present.

The job had almost convinced me that my children didn't deserve my time unless I was being paid for it, But one thing I know now is that taking care of your family is a job too. Waking up in the morning feeling rejuvenated and wanting to talk to my family and check in on their lives, reminded me of what really mattered. Most importantly, I realized that if I hadn't woken up to this problem, I might have lost sight of where my family was heading.

Closing Reflection

Leaving that job didn't just save me; it saved my family. It reminded me that stability doesn't come from a paycheck or a title, but it comes from the love and connection we nurture at home. Work may shape part of who we are, but it should never consume the whole of us. Choosing to heal meant choosing to show up for the people who matter most, and in that choice, I found a freedom no workplace could ever give me.

CHAPTER 7

A Call to Action for Leaders

Leaders hold enormous responsibility for the culture and health of their organizations. Creating a safe, thriving workplace doesn't happen by accident; it requires deliberate, consistent effort. Listening to your people is the first step. This isn't about empty gestures during exit interviews; it's about asking meaningful questions while staff are still present, engaged, and struggling. Leaders must create spaces where honesty is welcomed, experiences are validated, and problems are addressed head-on.

I've seen workplaces where leadership turned a blind eye, assuming resilience could fill every gap. I've also seen the difference in a workplace environment when a leader genuinely stepped in to understand the pressures that staff face. The message is clear—how leaders show up sets the tone for everyone else.

Walking in Their Shoes

One of the most overlooked responsibilities of leadership is truly understanding what staff experience daily. Too often, decisions are made from a distance, without a full grasp of the realities on the ground. Shadowing staff, attending meetings, or even spending a day in their role can provide insights no report or memo ever could.

When leaders take the time to witness challenges firsthand, it builds empathy, informs better decisions, and sends a powerful message that "I value your work enough to experience it myself." This level of engagement isn't a one-time gesture; it's ongoing, intentional, and consistent.

Training, Growth, and Support

Leadership isn't innate; it's learned and strengthened through training, reflection, and feedback. Organizations that invest in leadership development, communication skills, mental health awareness, and equity foster environments where staff feel supported and valued. Evaluations and surveys matter only if they're followed by action. Listening is only the first step because change must follow.

Self-care is equally important in a healthy workplace. Leaders who model boundaries and prioritize their own well-being show their teams that it's safe to do the same. A workforce that is mentally, physically, and emotionally supported is far better equipped to handle responsibilities effectively.

Recognition, Equity, and Accountability

Recognition and appreciation are powerful. Simply acknowledging contributions prevents staff from feeling invisible and fosters a sense of belonging. Equity ensures that promotions, opportunities, and resources are distributed fairly. Leaders must also be skilled in conflict resolution, stepping in early to mediate before issues escalate.

Accountability begins at the top. Leaders must welcome feedback, adjust practices when necessary, and model healthy behavior themselves. The impact of committed leadership ripples through the entire organization, influencing staff engagement, client outcomes, and workplace culture.

A Leader's Checklist for a Healthy, Thriving Workplace

1. **Listen to Your People** – Ask meaningful questions. Create safe spaces for honesty. Validate experiences and take action (Sinek, 2014; Harvard Business Review, 2016).

2. **Regular Training and Development** – Leaders and staff should engage in ongoing training on management, communication, mental health awareness, and equity (Lencioni, 2002; SHRM, 2022).

3. **Consistent Evaluations and Surveys** – Review results carefully and implement meaningful changes based on feedback (Gallup, 2023).

4. **Self-Care for Staff and Leaders** – Prioritize mental, physical, and emotional well-being for themselves and staff (NIOSH, 2021; Pink, 2011).

5. **Team Collaboration** – Promote strong teamwork, shared responsibilities, and mutual support (Coyle, 2018; Lencioni, 2002).

6. **Role Familiarity** – Shadow staff positions when possible to understand challenges firsthand (Sinek, 2014).

7. **Transparency in Decision-Making** – Clearly communicate the "why" behind organizational decisions (HBR, 2016; Coyle, 2018).

8. **Recognition and Appreciation** – Regularly acknowledge contributions and hard work (SHRM, 2022; Pink, 2011).

9. **Equity and Fairness** – Ensure opportunities, promotions, and resources are distributed without favoritism (Gallup, 2023).

10. **Conflict Resolution Skills** – Be prepared to mediate disputes before they escalate (Lencioni, 2002).

11. **Modeling Boundaries** – Lead by example in maintaining a healthy work-life balance (NIOSH, 2021; Pink, 2011).

12. **Accountability at the Top** – Welcome feedback and make changes when necessary (Sinek, 2014; HBR, 2016).

Reflection for Leaders

Think about the staff you lead. Are they showing up because they want to or because they feel obligated? Are your decisions informed by insight into their daily challenges or by reports and assumptions? Small, deliberate actions—listening, recognizing, supporting, and modeling healthy behavior—can change the trajectory of an organization.

Leadership isn't about power or authority; it's about responsibility. It's about shaping environments where people can thrive, innovate, and show up as their best selves. The health of your organization starts with the choices you make every day

References

Books

1. Sinek, S. (2014). *Leaders eat last: Why do some teams pull together and others don't*. Portfolio/Penguin.

2. Pink, D. H. (2011). *Drive: The surprising truth about what motivates us*. Riverhead Books.

3. Lencioni, P. (2002). *The five dysfunctions of a team: A leadership fable*. Jossey-Bass.

4. Coyle, D. (2018). *The culture code: The secrets of highly successful groups*. Bantam.

Articles & Reports

5. Harvard Business Review. (2016). *Why don't leaders listen?* HBR. Retrieved from https://hbr.org

6. Gallup. (2023). *State of the global workplace: 2023 report*. Gallup, Inc. Retrieved from https://www.gallup.com

7. Society for Human Resource Management (SHRM). (2022). *Employee recognition: How to motivate and retain employees*. Retrieved from https://www.shrm.org

Government / Nonprofit Resources

8. National Institute for Occupational Safety and Health (NIOSH). (2021). *Preventing occupational stress in the workplace.* Centers for Disease Control and Prevention. Retrieved from https://www.cdc.gov/niosh

9. Occupational Safety and Health Administration (OSHA). (2020). *Workplace stress.* U.S. Department of Labor. Retrieved from https://www.osha.gov

CHAPTER 8

Life Now

Today, my life looks different. I still work hard, but I work from a place of balance, not survival. I choose opportunities that align with my values, and I walk away from environments that compromise my peace.

I've learned to listen to my body when it tells me it needs rest. I've learned to trust my instincts when something feels off, and I've learned that my worth isn't tied to how much I produce or how much I can endure. Life now is not perfect, but it's mine, and it's built on the foundation of lessons learned through pain, resilience, and intentional healing.

The most surprising part? The more I've prioritized my own well-being, the more effective I've become in my work. Peace has made me more productive, not less. I no longer survive my work; I thrive in it. My rest is not a weakness; it's a superpower. Choosing peace doesn't make me soft; it makes me unstoppable. I honor my boundaries because they protect not just my energy but my purpose.

I no longer respond to phone calls after 8 p.m. When I'm off from work, I'm truly off. My availability is now clearly set. You can reach me between 8 a.m. and 4 p.m. because my mind and body can only operate this way without creating frustration and anxiety. I make sure my family sees me fully present beyond just completing necessities. I stay in environments that maintain my peace, and I recognize when I'm irritated or stressed or when I am approaching burnout.

I check in with myself regularly—noticing creeping headaches, low energy, or skipped meals. I've learned that I cannot overwork my mind or body anymore. Planning ahead with my family and friends has become essential for my well-being. The most important part of all this is recognizing when change is needed and making the effort, even in small steps. I reflect on how self-care truly looks and feels for me, and I write down the habits I want to leave behind versus those I want to create. Setting goals and checking in during the day ensures I stay aligned with my priorities.

I have no problem saying the word "**NO.**" It has taught me boundaries, stress relief, and self-respect. I am unapologetic about protecting my peace, and I will continue to honor these boundaries. My spiritual connection keeps me grounded, centered, and resilient, reminding me that peace, balance, and intentional living are not luxuries; they are necessities.

I also work for a family organization to which I'm related. I came in ready to help, carrying the weight of past experiences that made family work settings feel daunting. Those experiences left marks, but I've made a conscious choice to operate in a way that ensures we don't repeat the mistakes of my previous job. I focus on respect, account-ability, clear communication, which fosters diversity and equity, so no one feels trapped in patterns that once left me feeling hurt. This intentional approach allows me to contribute positively while protecting both myself and others.

By prioritizing well-being, fostering equity, and holding myself accountable, I've discovered that work can be a space of growth, not fear. Life now isn't perfect, but it's authentic, balanced, and empowered, and that is more than enough.

Reflection for the Reader:

- How would your "life now" look if you made decisions from a place of peace instead of fear?
- What boundaries would you set?
- What habits would you leave behind?
- What parts of yourself would you finally allow to flourish?

The life you want is possible, not because everything outside changes, but because your choices, your focus, and your care for yourself shift the world around you.

CONCLUSION

Healing Beyond the Hustle

Workplace trauma is real. Burnout is real. The harm that comes from toxic leadership, unbalanced workloads, and ignored mental health isn't just "part of the job;" it's a silent epidemic that reaches every corner of our lives.

But so is healing.

So is reclaiming your voice.

So is building a life and career that feeds your spirit instead of draining it.

This book isn't just my story; it's proof that transformation is possible. I've been in the place where exhaustion feels normal, where silence feels safer than speaking up, where you wonder if you'll ever find peace again. I've also made it to the other side, not because

I'm lucky, but because I made small, deliberate choices to protect my worth.

For the worker who feels stuck, you are not powerless. Every boundary you set, every conversation you initiate, and every moment you choose rest over hustle are acts of rebellion against systems that expect you to run yourself into the ground.

For the leader who wants to do better, it's not about grand gestures. It's about daily choices that show your people they matter. Listen more. Respond with empathy. Protect boundaries. Model balance. Remember that your actions or your silence have the power to harm or to heal.

The Bigger Picture

Healing beyond the hustle isn't just about leaving toxic workplaces. It's about changing the culture that normalizes harm in the first place. That starts with each of us, speaking up, supporting one another, and refusing to settle for less than respect.

- Your Next Step
- What's one small action you can take today to protect your peace?
- Who can you ask for support?
- What are you no longer willing to tolerate?

Start now. Every choice matters. Your life beyond the hustle begins with one deliberate step.

You deserve work that respects you, leaders who protect you, and a life that makes you feel alive, not just useful.

Here's my final word to you. Don't just survive your work. Create a life you don't need to recover from.

Personal Reflection

God gave me the wisdom to see, understand, and move differently. Protecting my peace and joy has become greater than anything else I could ask for. Along the way, I've learned the importance of being led into the right environments and surrounding myself with people who love and care for me. These people are not just family members, but they are individuals with good hearts and good intentions.

Reflection Page

Peace is my priority.

My rest is my power.

I choose balance over burnout.

About the Author

My name is LaToya Monroe-Love, and I am an advocate, author, mother, and community leader who is dedicated to helping others rise from the weight of trauma and reclaim their power. My background in behavioral science and years of experience supporting families and communities have shaped the way I see people, not just through their pain, but through their resilience.

Through my work in nonprofits, community programming, and faith-based outreach, I've had the privilege of supporting families impacted by violence, stress, and broken systems. I've coached youth in basketball, baseball, and cheerleading, and I've learned that the true strength of a community lies in the love and care we pour into one another.

I watched many of my co-workers be treated unfairly, often for things that should never have been questioned, and I realized how often these injustices go unnoticed, leaving families broken and unsure how to respond. That reality, along with the strength and sacrifices of my own family, who I believe suffered just as much as I did, helped me to write this book. To them, I owe both gratitude and an apology.

When I'm not working or writing, I enjoy listening to music, dancing, and spending time with my loved ones. I attend The Dwelling Place Church, and I continue to be a voice for those who are learning to speak again after being silenced.

Healing Beyond the Hustle is my testimony, my truth, and my gift to anyone walking the hard road back to themselves.

Author Bio

LaToya Monroe-Love is an advocate, leader, and mentor dedicated to helping individuals rise beyond burnout and reclaim balance in their lives. Drawing from her background in behavioral science and years of experience supporting families and communities, she combines professional insight with personal truth to inspire healing and growth.

She lives in Massachusetts with her family and enjoys helping others move **beyond the hustle** toward peace and purpose.